Important Disclaimer:

Do not use this product without physician approval. You should be in good physical condition and be able to participate in the exercise. Exerscribe is not a licensed medical care provider and represent that they have no expertise in diagnosing, examining, or treating medical conditions of any kind, or in determining the effect of any specific exercise on a medical condition. You should understand that when participating in any exercise or exercise program, there is the possibility of physical injury. If you engage in this exercise or exercise program, you agree that you do so at your own risk, are voluntarily participating in these activities, assume all risk of injury to yourself, and agree to release and discharge Exerscribe from any and all claims or causes of action, known or unknown, arising out of Exerscribe's negligence. Must be 18 years or older to use. Remove product immediately if you experience pain, discomfort, tingling, numbness, or change of skin color. Do not lift more than 20% of the MAXIMUM you can lift in one repetition without the bands. Exercise slowly and with control. Wear only at the top of your arms or top of your thighs. Do not wear for more than 20 minutes. Caution: May affect balance when worn on thighs. Not all exercises are suitable for everyone. Any exercise program including this one may result in injury. Consult with a medical professional before beginning this or any exercise program. The Creators, Producers, Participants, Affiliates and Distributors disclaim any liability or loss in conjunction with the information, exercises demonstrated, or instruction expressed herein.

No express or implied warranty (whether of merchantability, fitness for a particular purpose, or otherwise) or other guaranty is made as to the accuracy or completeness of any of the information or content contained in any of the pages in this web site or otherwise provided by Exerscribe, Inc. No responsibility is accepted and all responsibility is hereby disclaimed for any loss or damage suffered as a result of the use or misuse of any information or content or any reliance thereon. It is the responsibility of all users of this website to satisfy themselves as to the medical and physical condition of themselves and their clients in determining whether or not to use or adapt the information or content provided in each circumstance. Notwithstanding the medical or physical condition of each user, no responsibility or liability is accepted and all responsibility and liability is hereby disclaimed for any loss or damage suffered by any person as a result of the use or misuse of any of the information or content in this website, and any and all liability for incidental and consequential damages is hereby expressly excluded.

BFR BANDS
BLOOD FLOW RESTRICTION TRAINING

Who is BFR good for?

ANY BODY
—
EVERY BODY

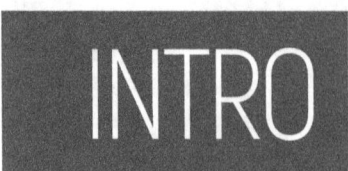

INTRO

When I first heard about blood flow restriction (BFR) training a few years ago, I thought 'no way, this can't be good for you.' But then I started seeing study after study publish on the safety and efficacy of BFR training in all populations. Men, women, young, old, athlete, injury rehab – all different types of people with different goals were benefitting from the use of BFR.

To date, there have been over 200 research studies to prove this training
methodology as an effective way to gain muscle, and get lean and tone. Not to mention that studies such as the one on Blood flow-restricted exercise in space suggests that "it is evident that this type of training could be applicable as an adjunct countermeasure to combat musculoskeletal and cardiovascular dysfunctions during missions beyond low-earth orbit."

Now, let's talk about why anyone would adopt BFR training. First off, learning how to get more from less is fundamentally human nature – I mean, who wouldn't want to get more muscle from their workout? BFR bands are a supplemental weightlifting tool that you can add to your existing routine that will allow you to lift less, but gain more muscle. Still skeptical? If you do Google Scholar search on BFR training you will find ample research on the topic.

As a technique of for weight training, BFR involves restricting venous blood flow from the muscle group that you are focusing on. The intent is to allow the venous blood to "pool" in the region of the body you're training (i.e. upper or lower limbs). By doing this, the body will naturally trigger several hormone responses that cause an anabolic push to the large fast twitch muscles. Because they are the largest muscle group, they are the most likely to gain mass and tone quickly.

BFR Training 101

The occlusion training bands should be applied right below the deltoid for the arms, or right below the hips on the quads. Also, they shouldn't feel terribly uncomfortable (you want to tighten to what feels like 70% pressure), and you shouldn't completely restrict all blood flow.

Most studies conducted on the value of occlusion training are similar to what you probably know as high-load training in terms of results. Studies show that, when compared to other types of training, occlusion-training results in greater development of muscle mass than without. BFR training also appears to increase muscle strength as well.

BFR Training Bands & How they work

How does it work? The premise is simple. When you workout using conventional methods, all of the metabolic byproducts of the workout move through and out of your body. With BFR training, the movement of the exertion hormones and byproducts are restricted from leaving the limbs, forcing them to pool in or near the trained region. By doing this, several things occur in your body. First, your body will interpret this occlusion and, in an attempt to compensate, will release more of the anabolic growth hormones. The production of protein is also increased. Restricting blood flow during your workout also has been shown to aid in the repair of cells and tissues that are broken down during the workout cycle.

Second, by restricting blood flow to the muscles that you are focusing on, the smaller slow twitch muscles fibers which rely on oxygen for energy starve out quickly, forcing the use and muscle damage of the fast twitch fibers - the fibers with the highest potential for growth. Type-II fast twitch muscle fibers are typically used during the final phase of a muscle contraction, not using oxygen, but by restricting blood flow the body must begin using the fast twitch fibers much sooner.

Occluded Blood Flow Technique

So, how should you train using this restrictive blood flow technique? Using your occlusion training bands, occlude the limbs of the area of the body you are focusing on. Tie it tight enough that it is mildly uncomfortable but not completely restricting all blood flow. This weightlifting technique is best used for a cycle of 4-8 weeks, or during the last week of each month as a de-load week to prevent overtraining.

BFR training is an extremely successful way to maximize your workout, allowing you to lift less weight and gain more muscle mass. It can be extremely painful and sometimes difficult, even when the load is light. It is an excellent way to grow and tone thigh, calf, and arm muscles. Studies have also shown that removing the occlusion during the workout to allow for a rush of the blood back to the muscle and the occluding it again does not produce a greater result, so it is better to leave the occlusion on during the entire workout.

The recommended load to lift during BFR is 20% of your maximum to achieve hypertrophy in the muscle and achieve the desired results. Considering several studies pertaining to this type of training, BFR training makes sense because major imbalances between muscle protein synthesis and muscle breakdown are the process that occurs during hypertrophy, the load lifted during the exercise is less important than what is actually occurring inside your body.

One other important key factor to consider is the release of various hormones as described previously. Several naturally occurring hormones are produced at an elevated rate during BFR. This elevation of hormone production has always been associated with acute resistance exercise routines with or without the restriction of blood flow, but the same product can be achieved with less workand to a higher degree.

BFR Training for Distant Muscle Groups

Muscle hypertrophy is what blood flow restricted studies have focused on. However, if you want to develop muscle groups apart from the occlusion sites like occlusion bands on upper arms, it may be good for you to use occlusion training.

This will be suitable if you want to increase your bench press strength and increase your chest muscle mass especially if you have an injury. Although it involves lighter weights, a new study has claimed that occlusion bench press helps to increase our muscle mass and strength if you have an injury or during inactivity.

Published in the Journal Clinical Physiology & Functional Imaging, the study examined the effect of restricting blood flow to the upper arm muscles especially during a low-intensity bench press workout. The study divided the volunteers into two groups.

One group was a control group while the other was a blood flow restricted group. For four weeks and six days every week, the two groups bench pressed 30 percent of their 1 repetition max (1RM) two times daily. There was a total of 75 repetitions during the workouts.

The group with the blood flow restricted bench pressed with elastic cuffs on both arms. It was noted that the pressure increase progressively on the two arms. External compression experienced an increase of 60 mmHg starting at 100 mmHg and ended at 160 mmHg.

The blood flow restricted group showed amazing results with an increase in muscle thickness experienced in the triceps, pectorals major ad an increase in the bench press strength. The triceps muscle thickness increased at a rate of 8 %, the pectorals major 16 % and the bench press increased to 6%. The control group 1RM bench decreased by 2%.

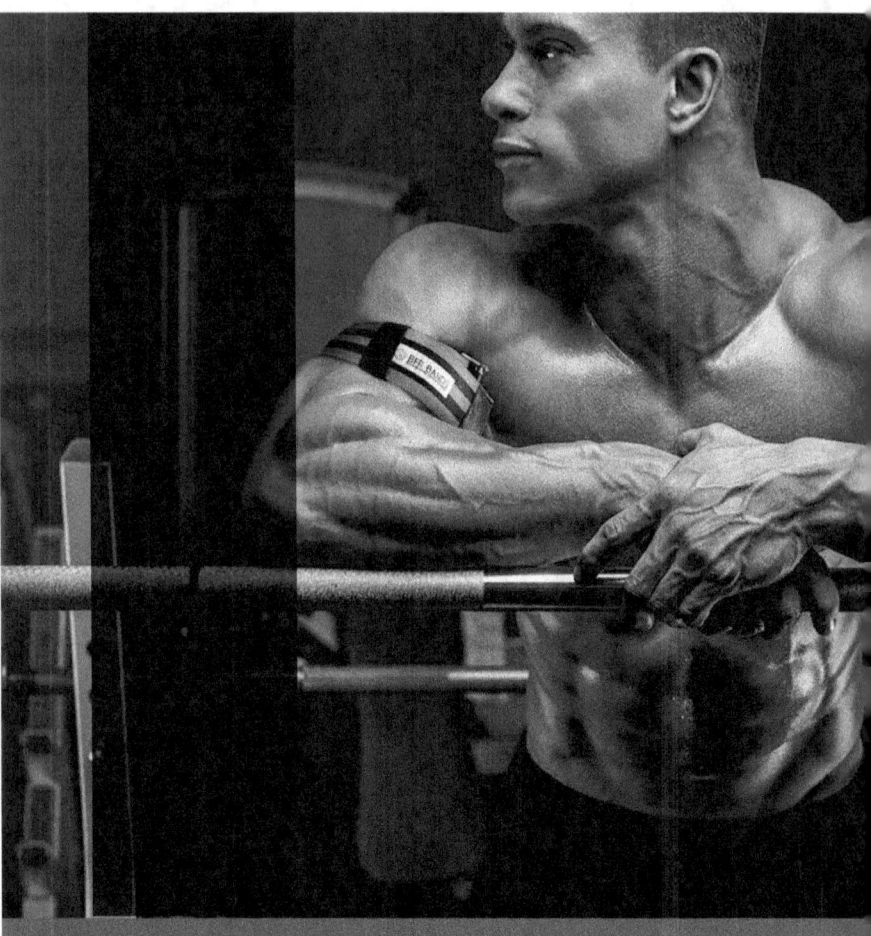

This study is applicable to individuals having an injury that affects their workout. The two groups in this study it should be noted were novices. With an injury, no advanced bench presser trains with 30% of his 1RM. When novices start their training, initial strength gains are neural. They get even better the movement pattern. Strength gain will take much longer because of the increased muscle mass.

Restricting blood flow to the upper arms while lifting light weights helps the bench presser to retain his or her muscle hypertrophy and also reach their maximum limit bench pressing strength. Those people who are mostly traveling and cannot easily find heavy weights can also benefit from this. By incorporating occlusion training into your workout, you can use light weights and still gain muscle mass.

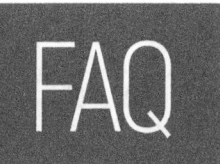

FAQ

Q. How do I know if the bands are too tight?

If you experience numbness or tingling, the bands are too tight and your workout should stop. On a perceived scale of tightness of 1-10 (10 feeling the tightest), the bands should feel like a 5 to a 7 (aka70% pressure). It's important to check this throughout the workout because you may be at optimal pressure near the beginning of the workout, but as the workout progresses and your "pump" increases so will the pressure in the bands.

Q. How tight exactly should the bands "feel" when I'm working out with them?

The bands should not actually feel as tight as you may think. The research suggests that you will attain the best results by tightening the bands to what feels like 70% pressure. If the bands do not feel tight enough initially, you may need to increase your training volume (i.e. 30-50 repetitions, 3-10 sets) and decrease your rest intervals (i.e. 20-30 seconds rest). Also, since everyone's body type, shape, and density is unique, some may find our PRO series bands or ELITE bands to be most suitable while others may find our CLASSIC or Rigid Edition models (which are rigid) to be more suitable. See the last question for the key differences between each model.

Q. Is Occlusion Training safe?

Yes. There are numerous research studies to support that blood flow occlusion training is safe and effective. One study even states that occlusion training is safer than traditional weight training which is performed with heavier loads. Since occlusion training is performed with light weights only (~20% of 1RM), it puts significantly less stress on the nervous system (brain) and body. Also, you are already performing "occlusion training" whenever you are performing weight training since the occlusion is happening internally.

Q. Who is Occlusion Training best for?

Occlusion training can be especially useful for those looking to gain lean muscle mass without lifting heavy weights. This includes women who prefer not to lift heavy weights (at least not all the time), men who need a "deload" week for active recovery from traditional training (good to do at least one week every month), those recovering from injuries, and those just seeking rapid gains in muscle size. Also, since blood flow restriction training creates a bolus of blood and nutrients which flood the muscle/joint, it is theorized that it strengthens tissues (i.e. ligaments and tendons). Stronger ligaments and tendons is great for injury prevention but also helps lower your brain's "threat" levels, which in turn makes your brain feel comfortable to increase your muscle strength contractile capabilities.

Q. How often should I perform Occlusion Training?

For most people, 2-3 days per week is sufficient. It is also something you can integrate into a current routine, such as on your rest days, as an active recovery week, or even at the end of your workout. The bands could even be worn on the legs while performing a light cardio routine for 20 minutes. With regard to aerobic activity, one study states "BFR aerobic (walking and cycling) exercise training methods have also recently emerged in an attempt to enhance cardiovascular endurance and functional task performance while incorporating minimal exercise intensity. Low-intensity BFR aerobic exercise [...] enhances muscle size and strength and simultaneously increases aerobic fitness."

Q. How many sets and repetitions should I be doing?

This all depends on the context of your goals, but generally you will see the best results performing 4-6 exercises for 3-10 sets each and 20-50 repetitions each. The weight used should of course be very light (only 20% of your 1 repetition maximum) and the rest period between sets should be short as well (20-30 seconds). Feel free to contact us anytime with questions.

Q. Where should I place the bands?

The BFR Bands can be placed on the upper arms (if training upper body) or upper legs if training lower body. Also, the bands do not have to directly occlude an area to provide benefit. For example, you will get the benefits of occlusion training for muscle groups like the chest and back when the bands are on the arms, even though they are not directly occluded.

Q. What is the difference between different versions of the bands?

CLASSIC Bands - just under 1 inch wide and made of a very rigid non-elastic material. These are great for a beginner to BFR training, and those with a body type that requires something more rigid.

ELITE Bands - 1.5 inches wide and made of a comfortable elastic material. These are great for the novice to BFR training, and those with a body type that requires something more comfortable. These are now thicker, longer (40 inches in length) and include a new marking system for increased precision and symmetry.

PRO Bands - 2 inches wide and made of an extra strong, durable elastic material. These are great for someone more advanced and those with more muscular body types. Because of the additional width, these can also work better the lower body. Our PRO BFR Bands LONG Edition may be necessary for those seeking even higher pressure. Also, our all new PRO-X Edition BFR Bands have a patented pullto- tighten system for easy one-handed operation, plus markings for tracking pressure, and training with symmetry and consistency.

Rigid Edition Bands - These come in two sizes. One size is for arms and is 18 inches long and the other is for legs and is 30 inches long. Both are 2 inches wide. These bands are rigid (no elasticity) and use a slim metal slider.These are most popular for those who want something rigid and prefer the metal slider instead of a buckle.

Double Wrap Bands - 3 inches wide and 42 inches long, most popular for legs and calves. With two portions of velcro, these bands are quick and easy to wrap up. The first portion of velcro helps you get the wrap started and held in place while the second portion of velcro holds the end in place.

QUAD Wrap Bands - 3 inches wide and 80 inches long, these bands are the most heavy duty leg wraps available. Equipped with a marking system so you can track pressure and train with symmetry as well as elastic loops to help you hold the band in place while tightening.

SLIDER SERIES Bands - These come as a bundle of 1.5 inch arm bands and 2 inch wide leg bands. They are very similar to our Rigid Edition BFR Bands in that they have velcro and slider (instead of buckle), however they do have some elasticity so they can flex with the muscle.

Conclusion

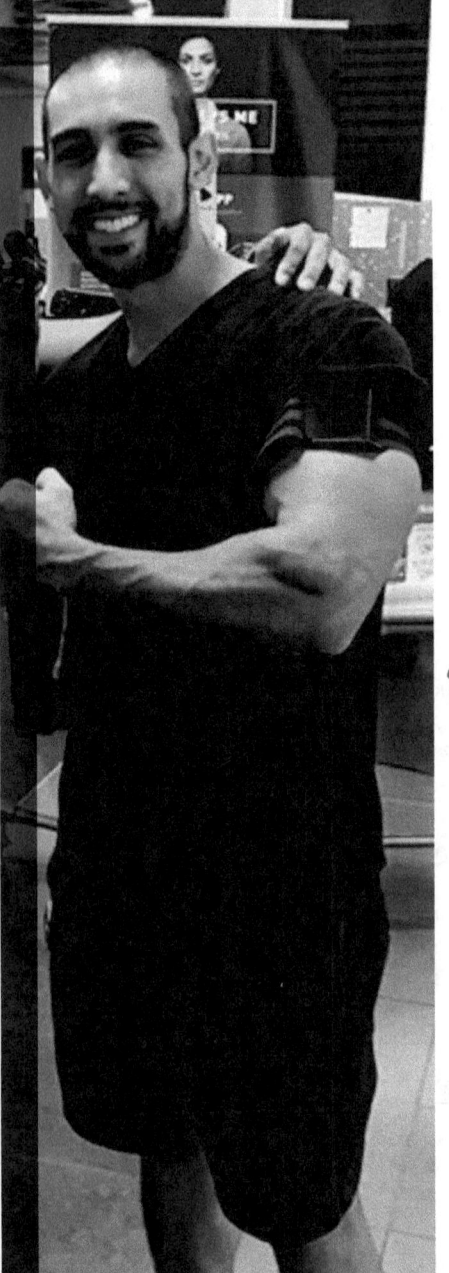

SO – what do we take from all of this?

Blood flow restriction can produce the same or better results with less weight. This type of exercise works great as a stand-alone or an adjunct to a traditional workout routine, and is a tool that should definitely be considered when trying to maximize gains.

Get after it,

Kusha Karvandi
PES, CES, CSCS

P.S. If you're still not convinced, check out the research studies in the References section at the end of this book.

Where to place the bands

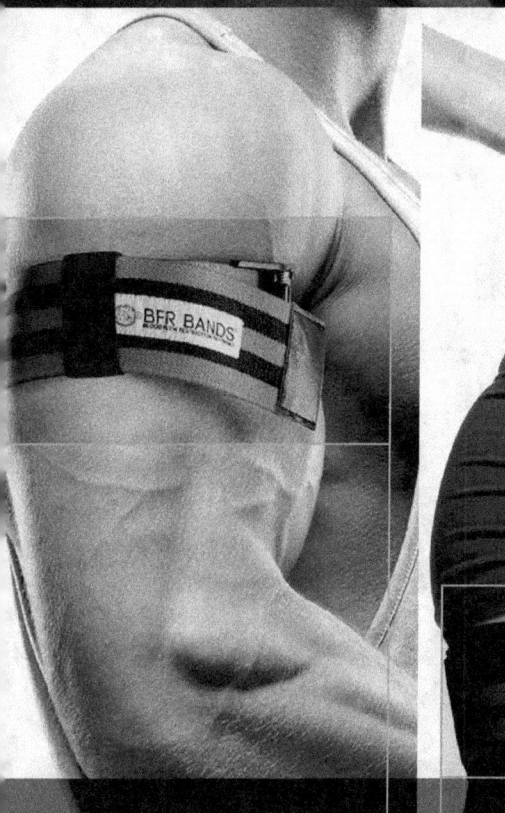

ARMS bands should be worn at the top of the arm
WHERE THE BICEPT MEETS THE DELTOID

LEGS bands should be worn at the top of the leg
JUST BELOW THE GLUTEAL FOLD

HOW TO STRAP UP

(All of Our Bands with This Style Buckle Should be Threaded This Way)

STEP 1

STEP 2

STEP 4

(You can double, triple, or quadruple wrap as necessary to achieve desired level of tightness)

STEP 3

Video Quick Start Guides

Classic Elite, & PRO BFR Bands Quick Start Guide: https://www.amazon.com/dp/B075D1ZK1F

PRO-X BFR Bands Quick Start Guide: https://www.amazon.com/dp/B07672T2L1

PRO-X BFR Bands & PRO BFR Bands Comparison: https://www.amazon.com/dp/B077XBTW8J

Rigid Edition BFR Bands Arms Quick Start Guide: https://www.amazon.com/dp/B076FRG3G1

Rigid Edition BFR Bands Legs Quick Start Guide: https://www.amazon.com/dp/B076FRP517

Double Wrap BFR Bands Quick Start Guide: https://www.amazon.com/dp/B076FRN15B

QUAD Wrap BFR Bands Quick Start Guide: https://www.amazon.com/dp/B076DXMV6S

BFR Knee Wraps Quick Start Guide: https://www.amazon.com/dp/B076DYDXVK

BFR Wrist Wraps Quick Start Guide: https://www.amazon.com/dp/B075MZQFXR

Slider Series BFR Bands Quick Start Guide: https://www.amazon.com/dp/B078XSHVKD

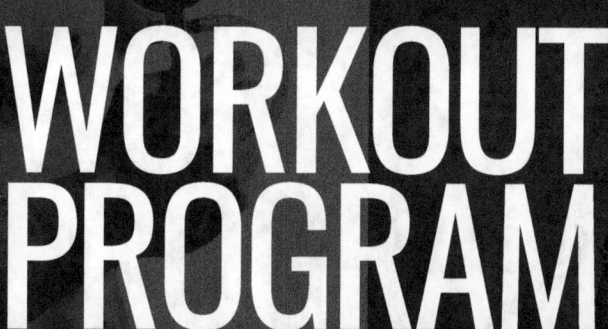

WORKOUT PROGRAM

Here are examples of workouts you can do for each muscle group.

*Note: When you see the letters A and B associated with exercises (i.e. Chest 2A and Chest 2B) it means they should be performed back-to-back as a superset.

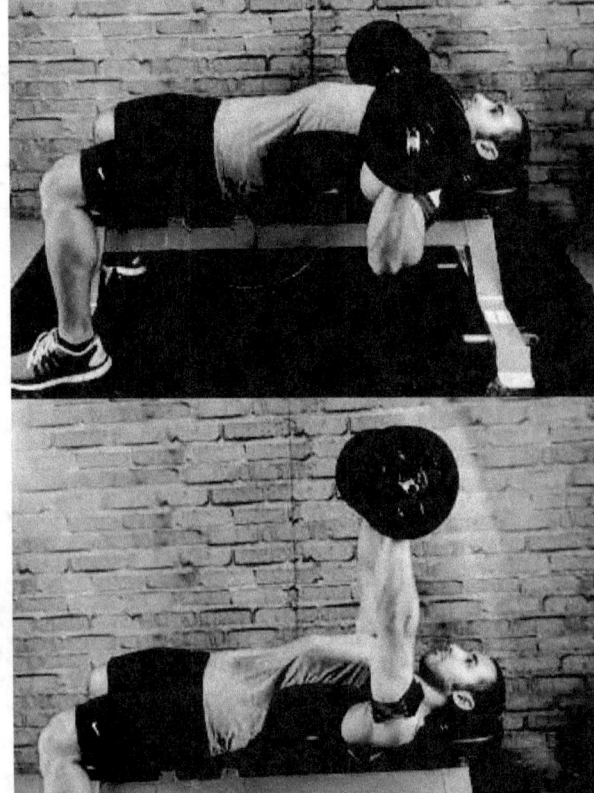

CHEST

1 Biohacking Muscle
With Blood Flow Restriction Training

DUMBBELL FLAT CHEST PRESS

Reps: **30, 15, 15, 15**
Sets: **4**
Rest: **30 seconds**

1

2

Biohacking Muscle
With Blood Flow Restriction Training

DUMBBELL INCLINE CHEST PRESS

Reps: **30, 15, 15, 15**
Sets: **4**
Rest: **30 seconds**

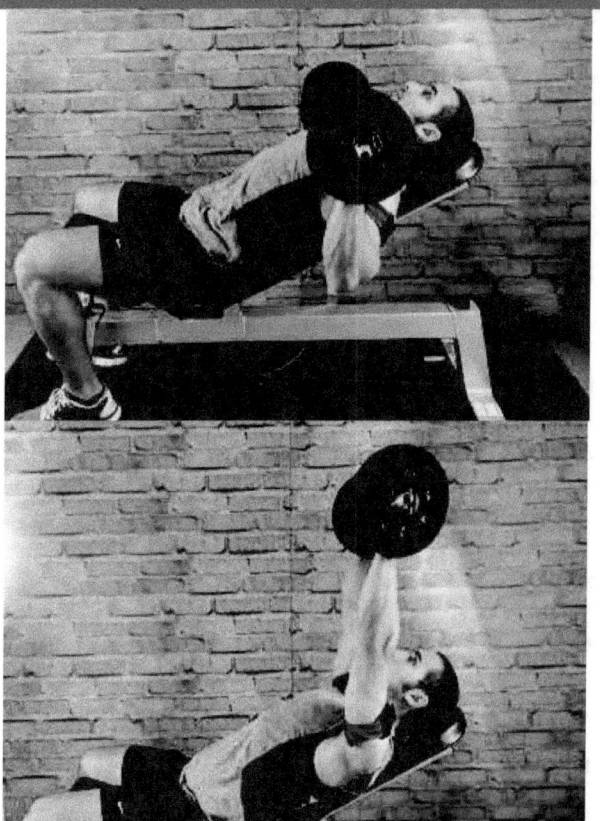

1

2

2B Biohacking Muscle
With Blood Flow Restriction Training

PUSHUPS

Reps: **30, 15, 15, 15**
Sets: **4**
Rest: **30 seconds**

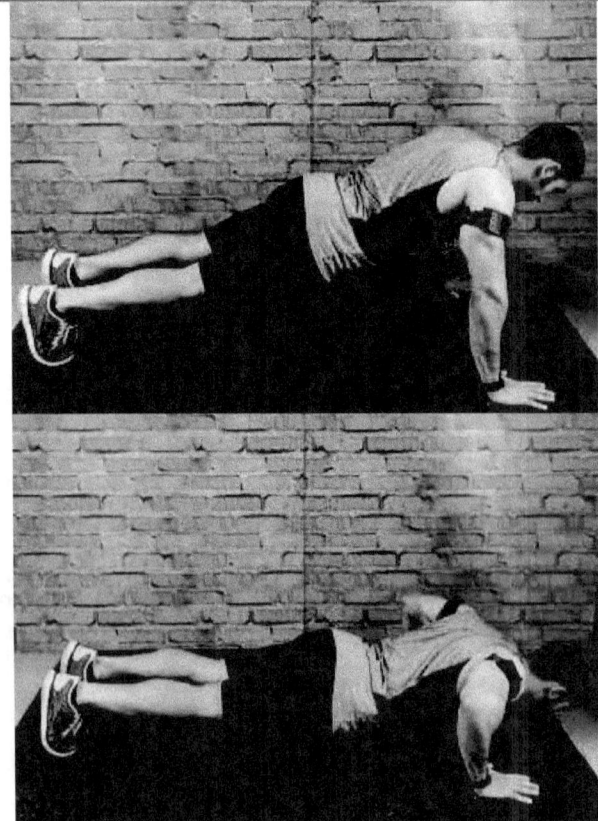

1

2

Biohacking Muscle
With Blood Flow Restriction Training

HAMMER CURLS

Reps: 30, 15, 15, 15
Sets: **3**
Rest: **NONE**

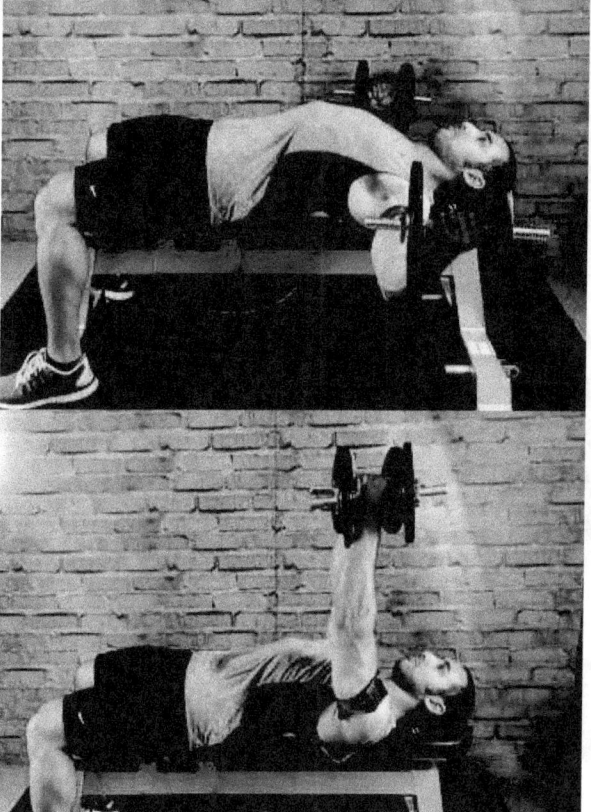

1

2

1 Biohacking Muscle
With Blood Flow Restriction Training

DUMBBELL BENT OVER ROW

Reps: **30, 15, 15, 15**
Sets: **4**
Rest: **30 seconds**

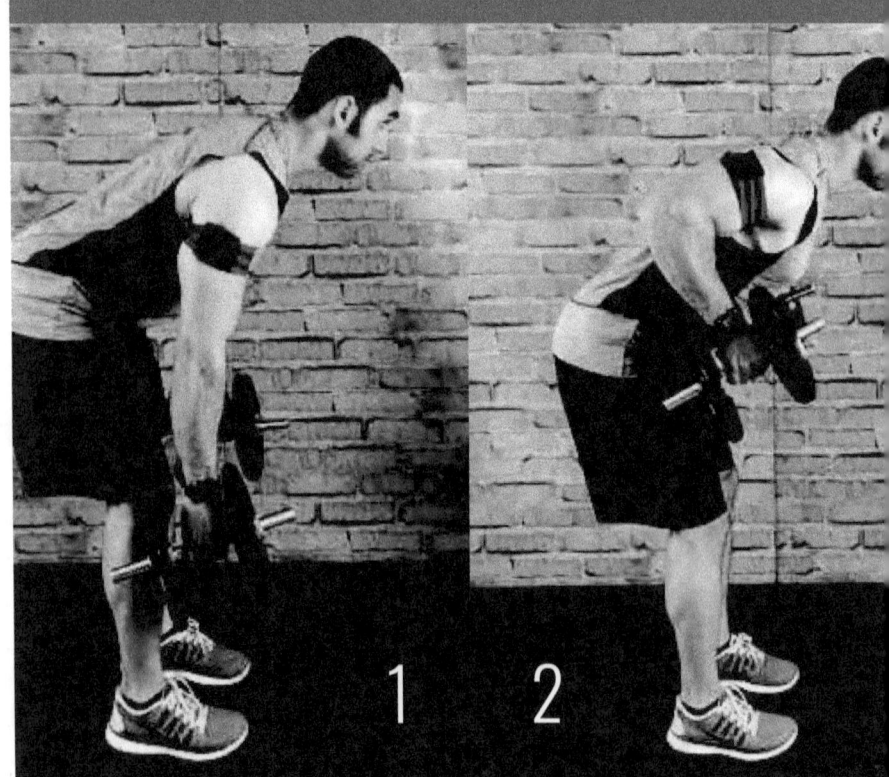

Biohacking Muscle
With Blood Flow Restriction Training

ONE ARM ROW

Reps: **30, 15, 15, 15**
Sets: **4**
Rest: **30 seconds**

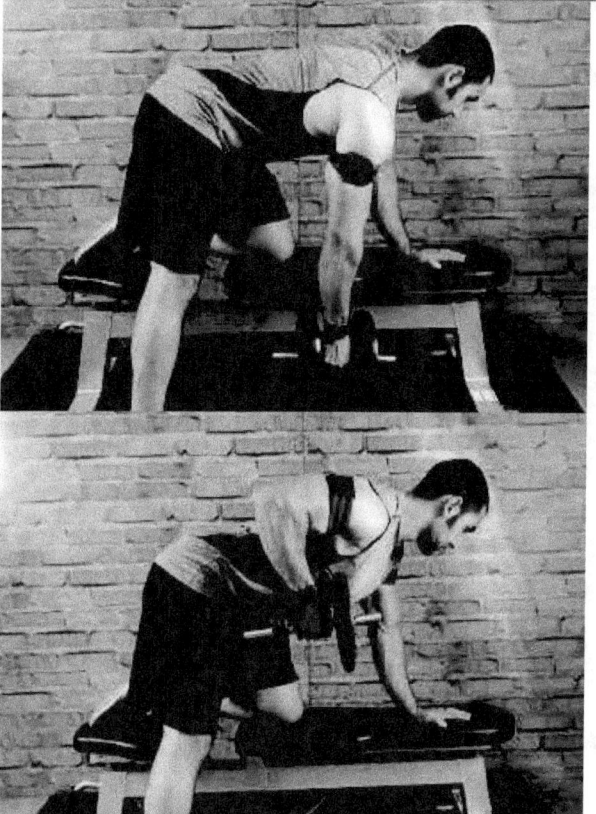

1

2

BAND WIDE ROWS

Reps: **30, 15, 15, 15**
Sets: **4**
Rest: **30 seconds**

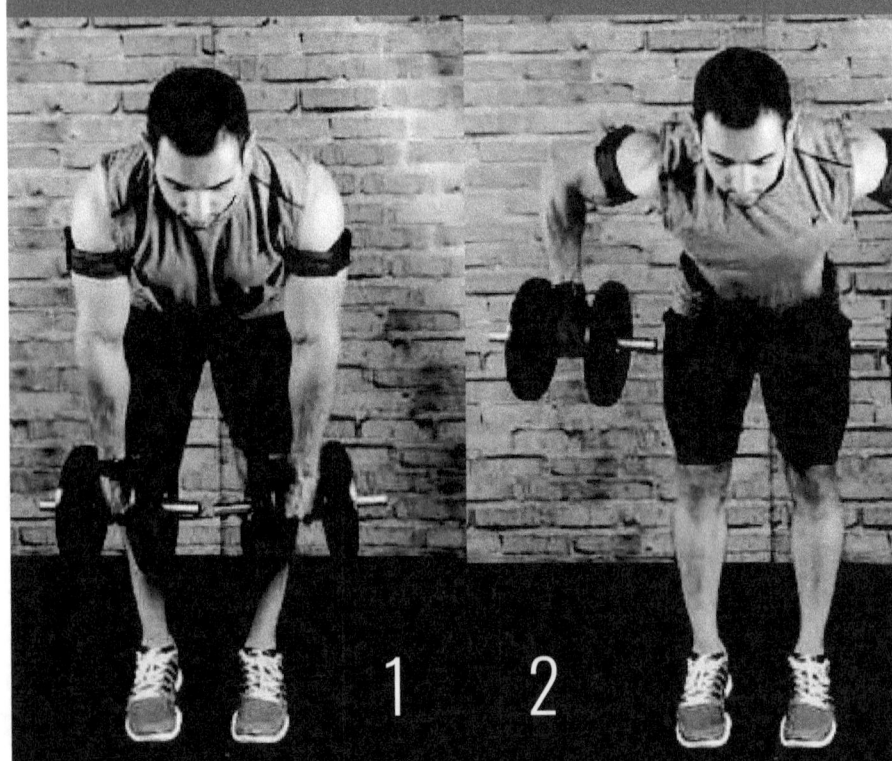

Biohacking Muscle
With Blood Flow Restriction Training

INCLINE BENCH ROW

Reps: **Drop sets - 20 (20% of 1RM), 25 (15% of 1RM), 30 (10% of 1RM)**

Sets: **3**

Rest: **NONE**

Notes: Perform these as drop sets, using 20% of 1RM (Rep Max) on the first set,
then immediately to 25 reps with 15% of 1RM, and then immediately to
30 reps with 10% of 1RM.

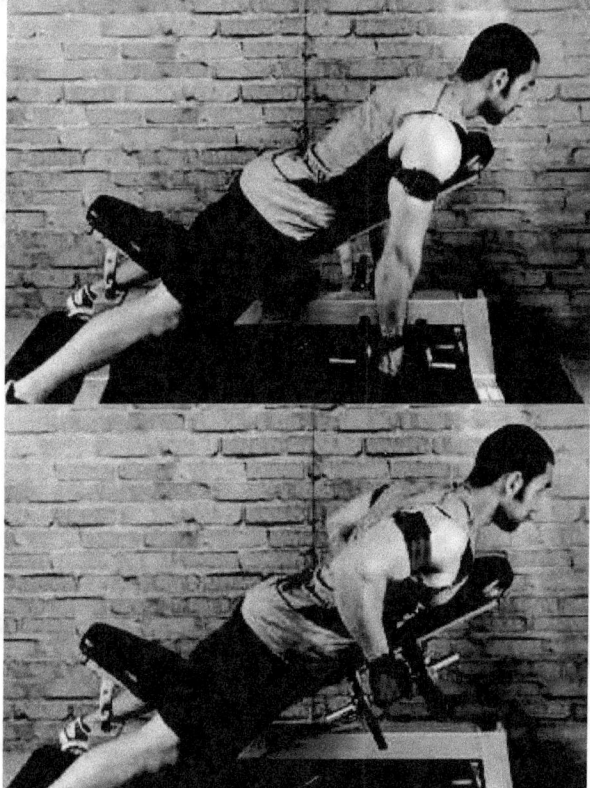

1

2

1 Biohacking Muscle
With Blood Flow Restriction Training

DUMBBELL CURLS

Reps: **30, 15, 15, 15**
Sets: **4**
Rest: **30 seconds**

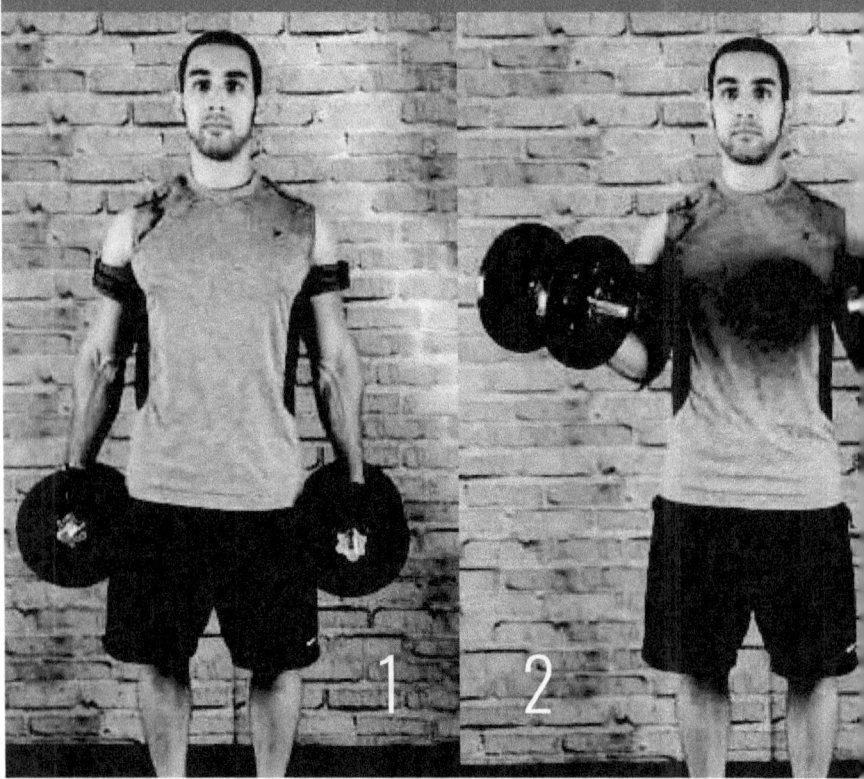

Biohacking Muscle
With Blood Flow Restriction Training

DUMBBELL KICKBACKS

Reps: **30, 15, 15, 15**
Sets: **4**
Rest: **30 seconds**

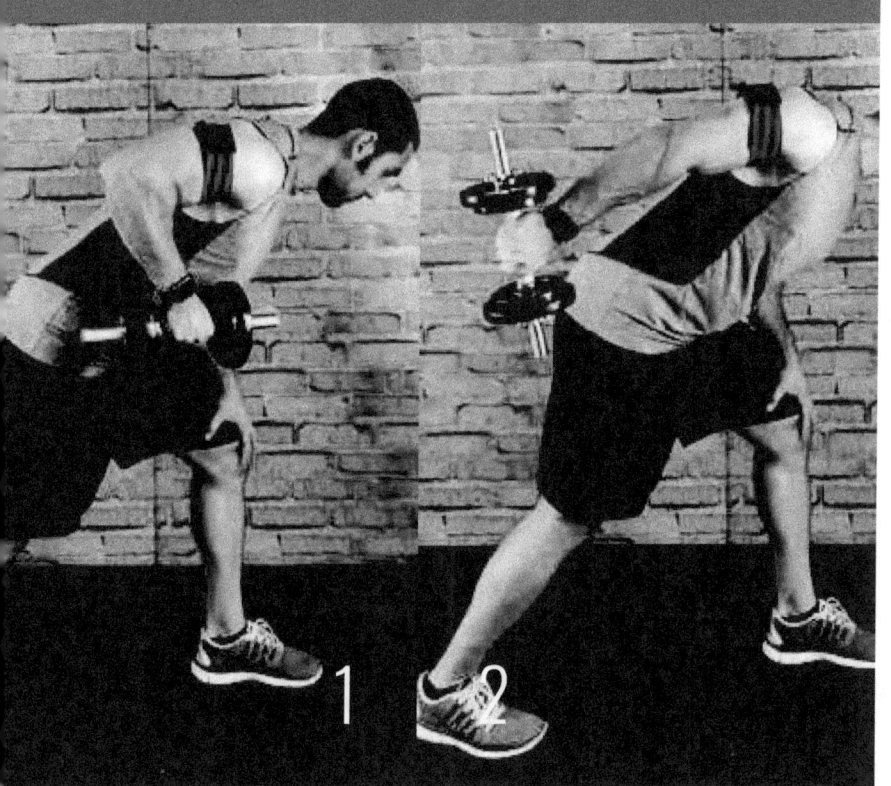

1   2

ARMS
3A Biohacking Muscle
With Blood Flow Restriction Training

WIDE CURLS

Reps: **30, 15, 15, 15**
Sets: **4**
Rest: **30 seconds**

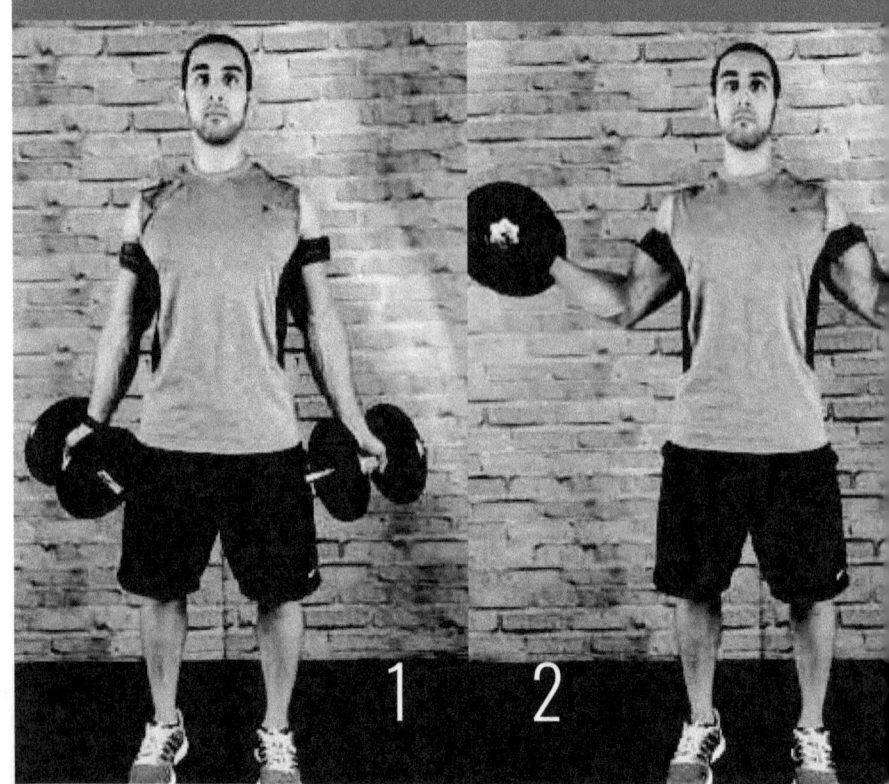

Biohacking Muscle
With Blood Flow Restriction Training

INCLINE BENCH ROW

Reps: **Drop sets - 20 (20% of 1RM), 25 (15% of 1RM), 30 (10% of 1RM)**

Sets: **3**

Rest: **NONE**

Notes: Perform these as drop sets, using 20% of 1RM (Rep Max) on the first set, then immediately to 25 reps with 15% of 1RM, and then immediately to 30 reps with 10% of 1RM.

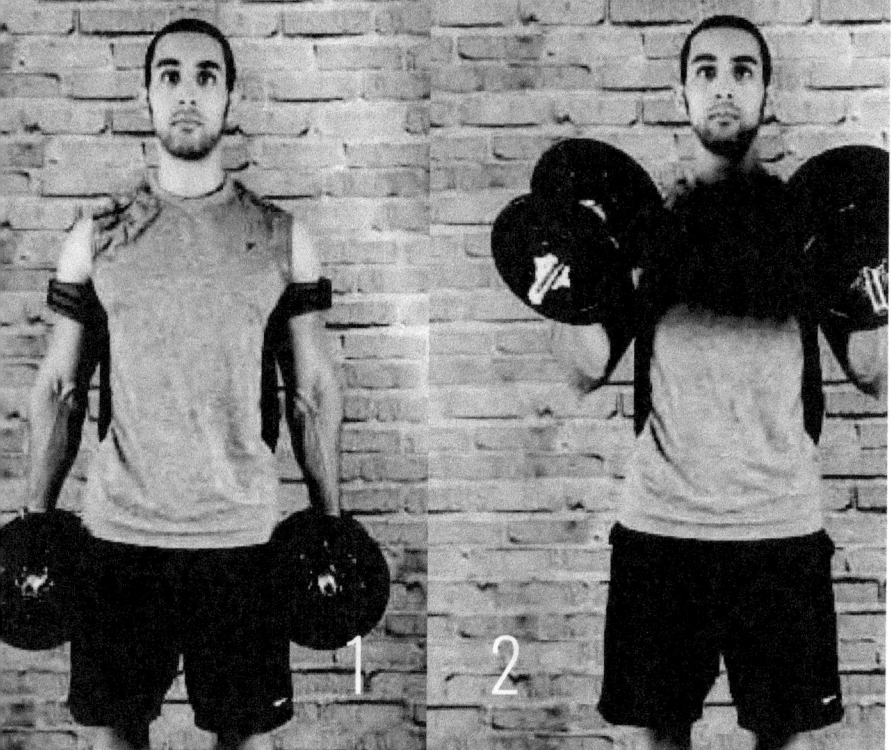

4A Biohacking Muscle
With Blood Flow Restriction Training

OVERHEAD DUMBBELL EXTENSION

Reps: **30, 15, 15, 15**
Sets: **4**
Rest: **30 seconds**

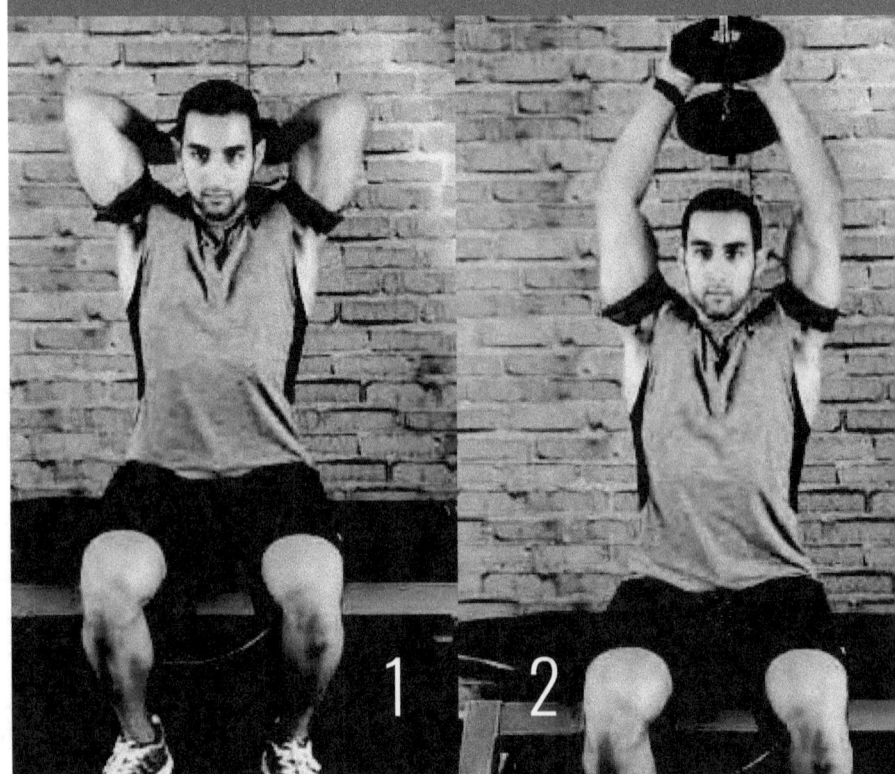

Biohacking Muscle
With Blood Flow Restriction Training

BENCH DIPS

Reps: **30, 15, 15, 15**
Sets: **4**
Rest: **30 seconds**

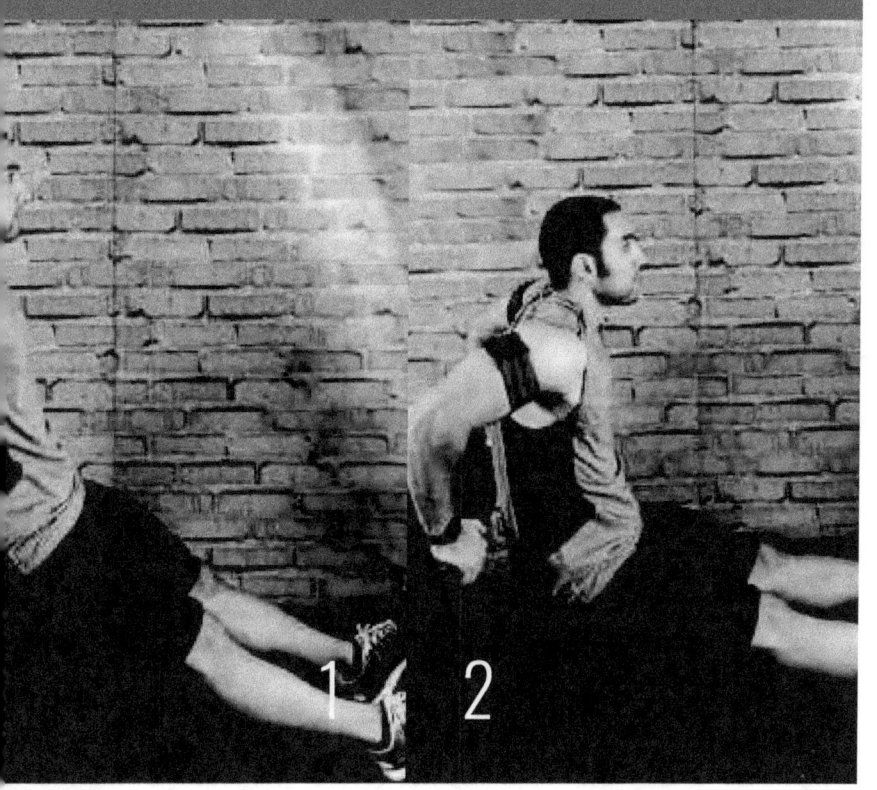

1

Biohacking Muscle
With Blood Flow Restriction Training

DUMBBELL SHOULDER PRESS

Reps: **30, 15, 15, 15**
Sets: **4**
Rest: **30 seconds**

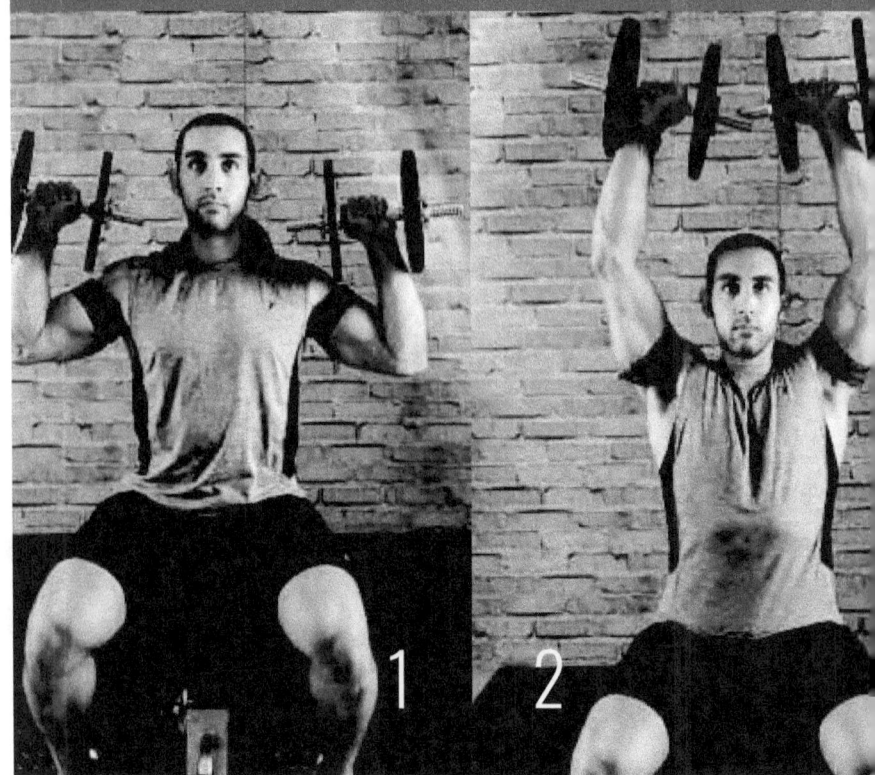

Biohacking Muscle
With Blood Flow Restriction Training

UPRIGHT ROW

Reps: **30, 15, 15, 15**
Sets: **4**
Rest: **30 seconds**

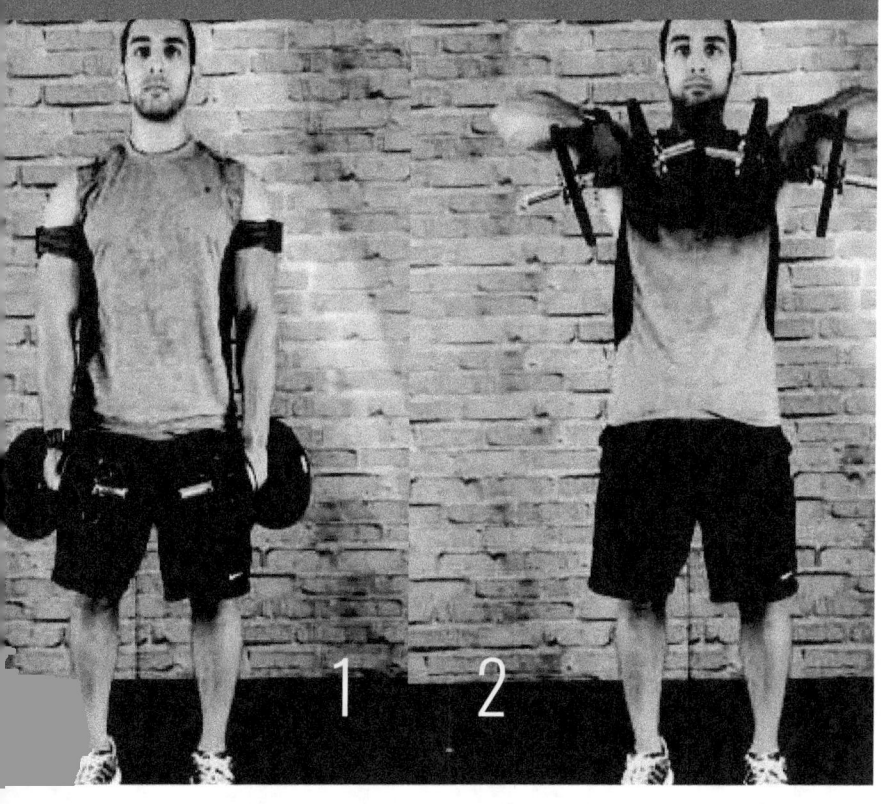

2B Biohacking Muscle
With Blood Flow Restriction Training

DUMBBELL SCAPTION

Reps: **30, 15, 15, 15**
Sets: **4**
Rest: **30 seconds**

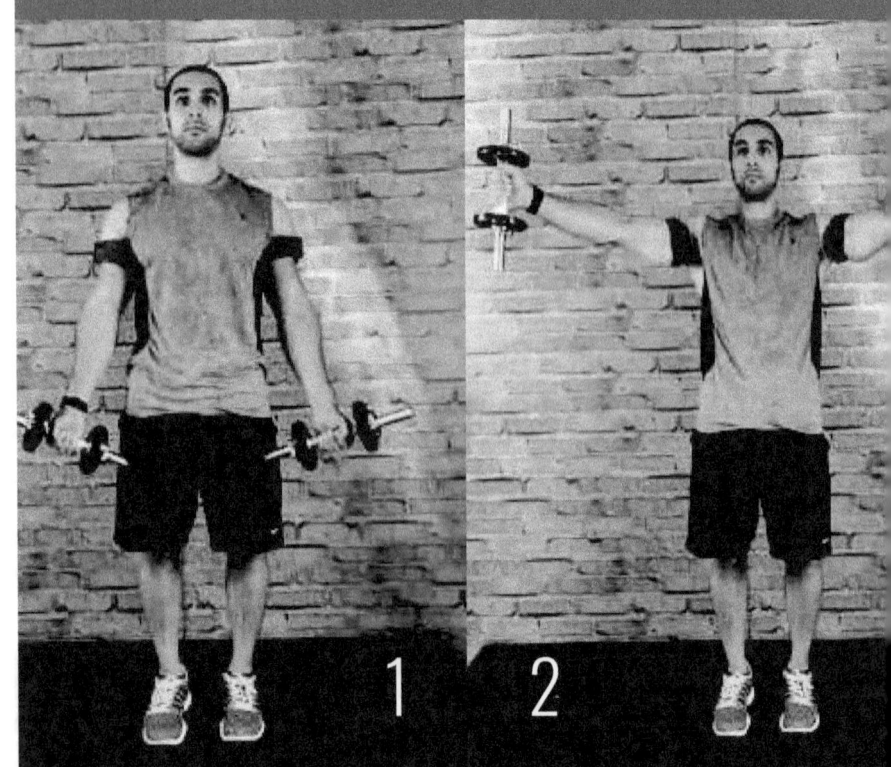

Biohacking Muscle
With Blood Flow Restriction Training

REAR DELT FLYES

Reps: **Drop sets - 20 (20% of 1RM), 25 (15% of 1RM), 30 (10% of 1RM)**

Sets: **3**

Rest: **NONE**

Notes: Perform these as drop sets, using 20% of 1RM (Rep Max) on the first set, then immediately to 25 reps with 15% of 1RM, and then immediately to 30 reps with 10% of 1RM.

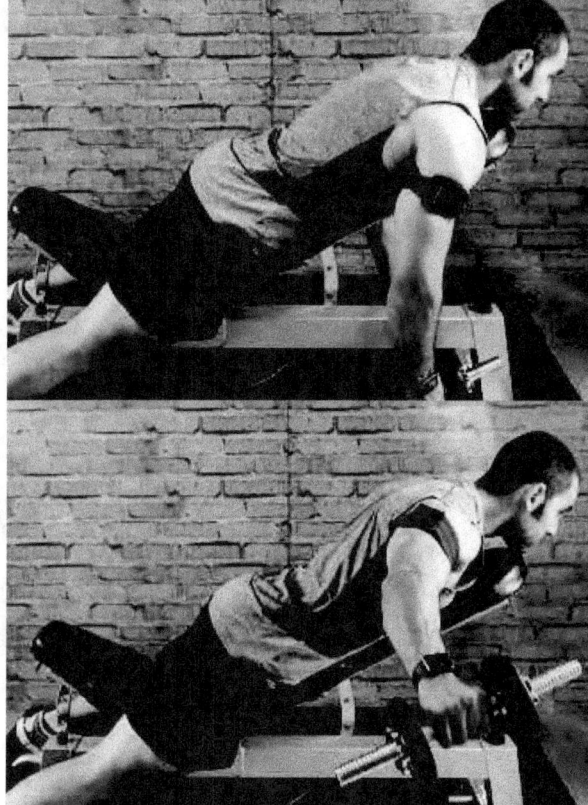

1

2

Biohacking Muscle
With Blood Flow Restriction Training

DUMBBELL SQUAT

Reps: **30, 15, 15, 15**
Sets: **4**
Rest: **30 seconds**

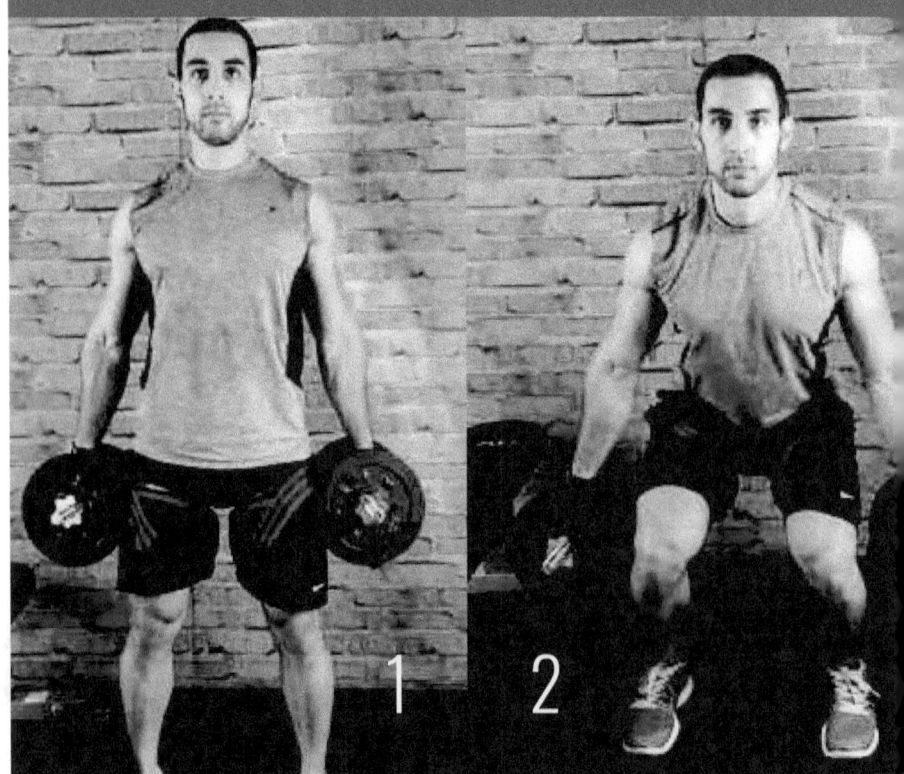

Biohacking Muscle
With Blood Flow Restriction Training

BULGARIAN SPLIT SQUAT

Reps: **30, 15, 15, 15**
Sets: **4**
Rest: **30 seconds**

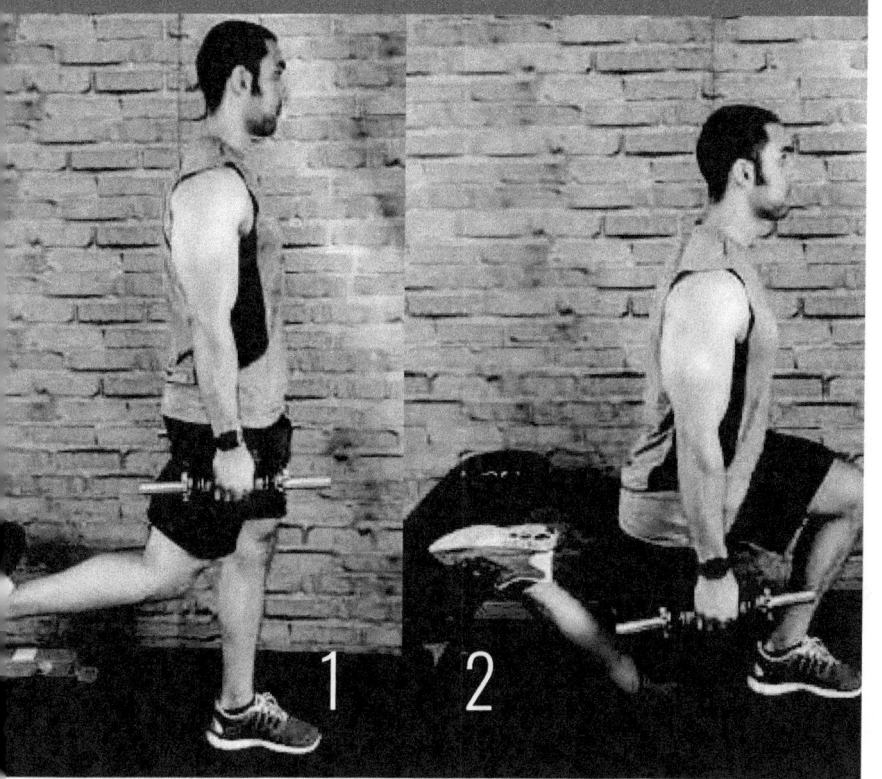

2B Biohacking Muscle
With Blood Flow Restriction Training

STEP UP TO BALANCE

Reps: **30, 15, 15, 15**
Sets: **4**
Rest: **30 seconds**

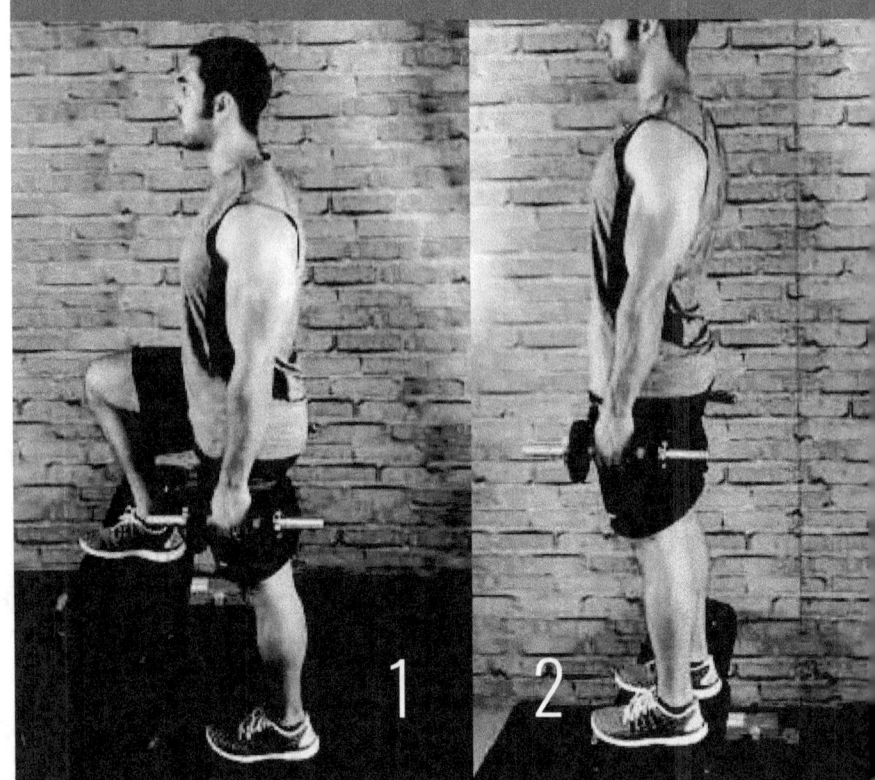

Biohacking Muscle
With Blood Flow Restriction Training

STRAIGHT LEG DEADLIFT

Reps: **Drop sets - 20 (20% of 1RM), 25 (15% of 1RM), 30 (10% of 1RM)**

Sets: **3**

Rest: **NONE**

Notes: Perform these as drop sets, using 20% of 1RM (Rep Max) on the first set, then immediately to 25 reps with 15% of 1RM, and then immediately to 30 reps with 10% of 1RM.

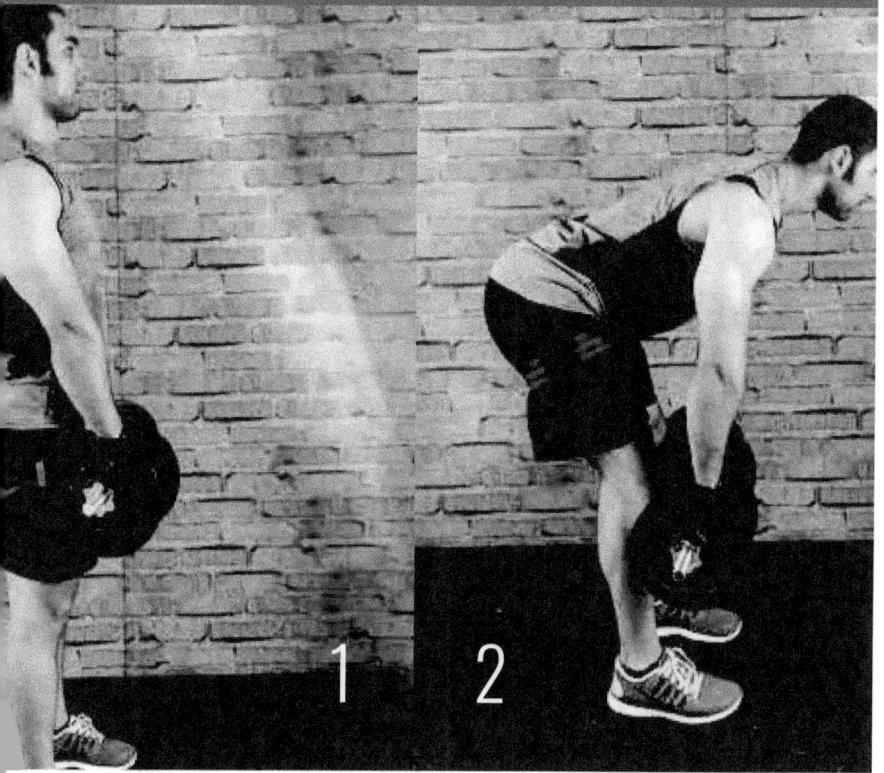

LEGS

4 Biohacking Muscle
With Blood Flow Restriction Training

CALF RAISE

Reps: **30, 15, 15, 15**
Sets: **4**
Rest: **30 seconds**

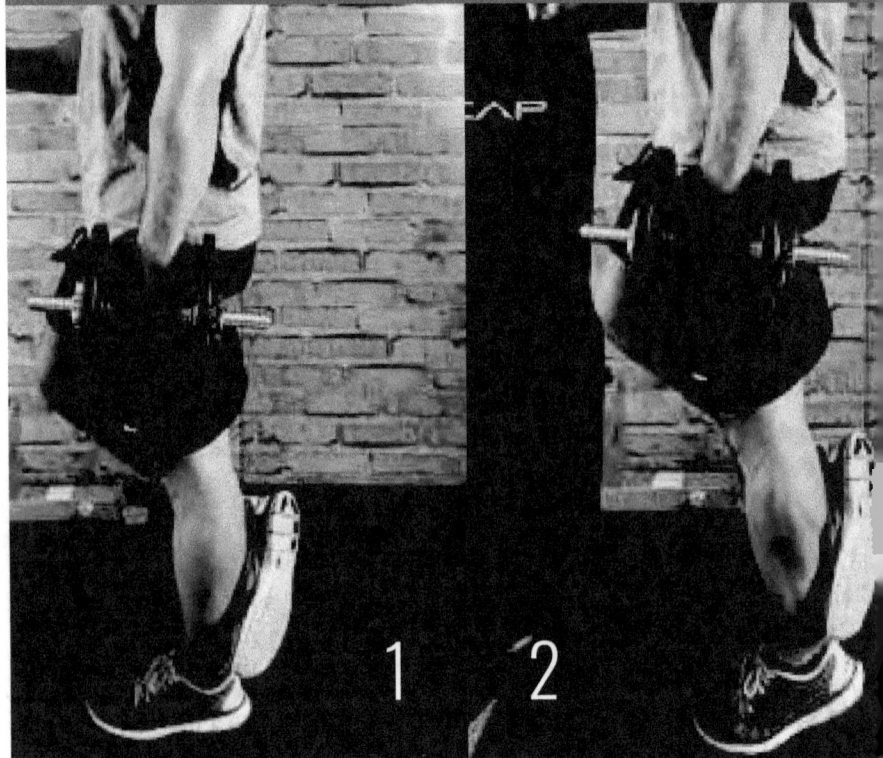

Biohacking Muscle
With Blood Flow Restriction Training

CRUNCHES

Reps: **30, 15, 15, 15**
Sets: **4**
Rest: **30 seconds**

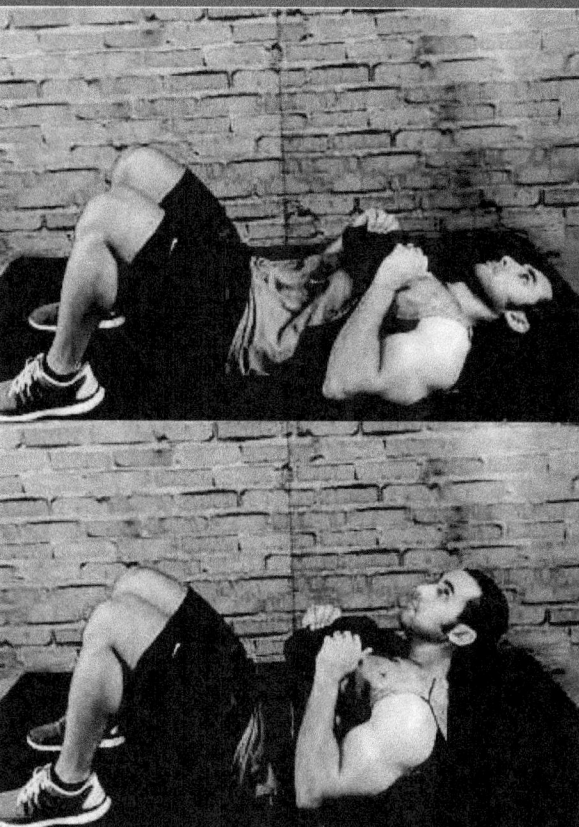

Biohacking Muscle
With Blood Flow Restriction Training

REVERSE CRUNCH

Reps: **30, 15, 15, 15**
Sets: **4**
Rest: **30 seconds**

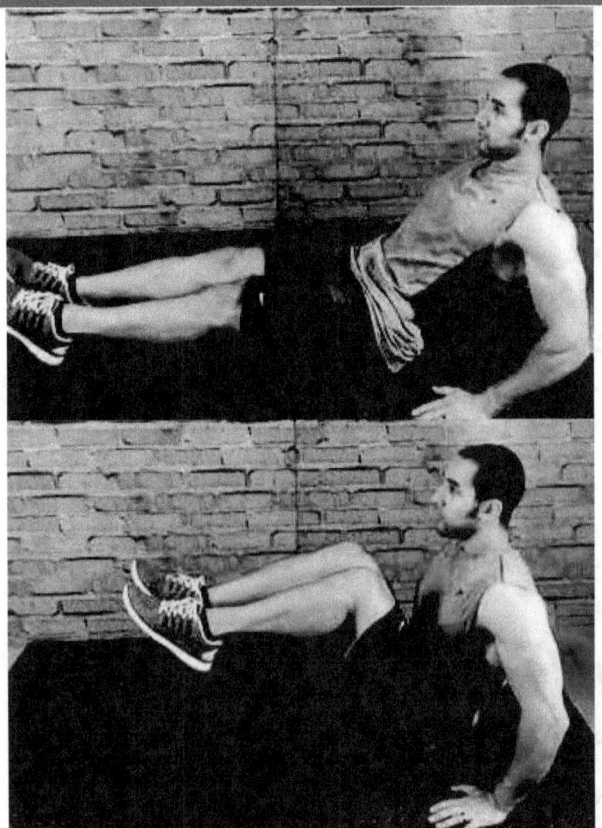

1

2

ABS

2B Biohacking Muscle
With Blood Flow Restriction Training

RUSSIAN TWIST

Reps: **30, 15, 15, 15**
Sets: **4**
Rest: **30 seconds**

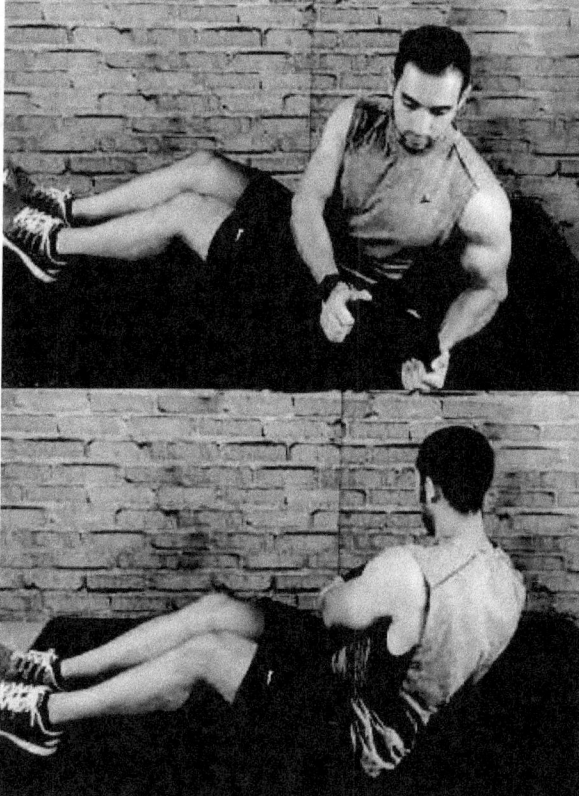

1

2

References

Abe T, Kearns C, Sato Y. Muscle size and strength are increased following walk training with restricted venous blood flow from the leg muscle, Kaatsu-walk training. J Appl Physiol 2006; 100 : 1460 – 1466.

Anderson JE. A role for nitric oxide in muscle repair: Nitric oxidemediated activation of muscle satellite cells . Mol Biol Cell 2000; 11 : 1859 – 1874.

Anderson JE, Wozniak AC. Satellite cell activation on fibers: modeling events in vivo – an invited review. Can J Physiol Pharmacol 2004 ; 82 : 300 – 310.

Dodd S, Hain B, Judge A. Hsp70 prevents disuse muscle atrophy in senescent rats. Biogerontology 2008.

Drummond MJ, Fujita S, Takashi A, Dreyer HC, Volpi E, Rasmussen BB. Human muscle gene expression following resistance exercise and blood flow restriction. Med Sci Sports Exerc 2008; 40 : 691 – 698.

Ehrnborg C, Rosen T. Physiological and pharmacological basis for the ergogenic effects of growth hormone in elite sports. Asian J Androl 2008; 10 : 373 – 383.

Fujita S, Abe T, Drummond MJ, Cadenas JG, Dreyer HC, Sato Y, Volpi E, Rasmussen BB. Blood flow restriction during low-intensity resistance exercise increases S6K1 phosphorylation and muscle protein synthesis. J Appl Physiol 2007; 103 : 903 – 910.

Gentil P, Oliveira E, Bottaro M. Time under tension and blood lactate response during four different resistance training methods . J Physiol Anthropol 2006; 25 : 339 – 344.

Gosselink KL, Grindeland RE, Roy RR, Zhong H, Bigbee AJ, Grossman EJ, Edgerton VR. Skeletal muscle afferent regulation of bioassayable growth hormone in the rat pituitary. J Appl Physiol 1998 ; 84 :1425 – 1430.

Grounds MD, Yablonka-Reuveni Z. Molecular and cell biology of skeletal muscle regeneration. Mol Cell Biol Hum Dis Ser 1993; 3 : 210 – 256

Idstrom JP, Subramanian VH, Chance B, Schersten T, Bylund-Fellenius AC. Energy metabolism in relation to oxygen supply in contracting rat skeletal muscle. Fed Proc 1986 ; 45 : 2937 – 2941.

Iida H, Kurano M, Takano H, Kubota N, Morita T, Meguro K, Sato Y, Abe T, Yamazaki Y, Uno K, Takenaka K, Hirose K, Nakajima T. Hemodynamic and neurohumoral responses to the restriction of femoral blood flow by KAATSU in healthy subjects. Eur J Appl Physiol 2007; 100 : 275 – 285.

References (cont)

Katz A, Sahlin K. Effect of decreased oxygen availability on NADH and lactate contents in human skeletal muscle during exercise. Acta Physiol Scand 1987; 131 : 119 – 127.

Kawada S, Ishii N. Changes in skeletal muscle size, fiber-type composition and capillary supply after chronic venous occlusion in rats. Acta Physiol Scand 2007; 192 : 541 – 549.

Kawada S, Ishii N. Skeletal muscle hypertrophy after chronic restriction of venous blood flow in rats. Med Sci Sports Exerc 2005; 37 : 1144 – 1150.

Kawada S, Tachi C, Ishii N. Content and localization of myostatin in mouse skeletal muscles during aging, mechanical unloading and reloading. J Muscle Res Cell Motil 2001; 22 : 627 – 633.

Kraemer WJ, Adams K, Cafarelli E, Dudley GA, Dooly C, Feigenbaum MS, Fleck SJ, Franklin B, Fry AC, Hoff man JR, Newton RU, Potteiger J, Stone MH, Ratamess NA, Triplett-McBride T. American College of Sports Medicine position stand. Progression models in resistance training for healthy adults. Med Sci Sports Exerc 2002; 34 : 364 – 380.

Kraemer WJ , Gordon SE , Fleck SJ , Marchitelli LJ , Mello R , Dziados JE, Friedl K, Harman E , Maresh C, Fry AC. Endogenous anabolic hormonal and growth factor responses to heavy resistance exercise in males and females. Int J Sports Med 1991; 12 : 228 – 235.

Kraemer WJ, Marchitelli L, Gordon SE, Harman E, Dziados JE, Mello R, Frykman P, McCurry D, Fleck SJ. Hormonal and growth factor responses to heavy resistance exercise protocols. J Appl Physiol 1990; 69 : 1442 –1450.

Loenneke, J., Wilson, J., Wilson, G., Pujol, T., & Bemben, M. (2011). Potential safety issues with blood flow restriction training. Scandinavian Journal of Medicine & Science in Sports, 510-518.

Loenneke, J., Wilson, G., & Wilson, J. (2009). A Mechanistic Approach to Blood Flow Occlusion. International Journal of Sports Medicine Int J Sports Med, 1-4.

McCroskery S, Thomas M, Maxwell L, Sharma M, Kambadur R. Myostatin negatively regulates satellite cell activation and self-renewal. J Cell Biol 2003; 162 : 1135 – 1147. McPherron AC, Lawler AM, Lee SJ. Regulation of skeletal muscle mass in mice by a new TGF-beta superfamily member. Nature 1997; 387 : 83 – 90.

McPherron AC, Lee SJ. Double muscling in cattle due to mutations in the myostatin gene. Proc Natl Acad Sci USA 1997; 94 : 12457 – 12461.

Mesires NT, Doumit ME. Satellite cell proliferation and differentiation during postnatal growth of porcine skeletal muscle. Am J Physiol Cell Physiol 2002; 282 : C899 – 906.

References (cont)

Moritani T, Muro M, Nagata A. Intramuscular and surface electromyogram changes during muscle fatigue. J Appl Physiol 1986; 60 : 1179 – 1185.

Moritani T, Sherman WM, Shibata M, Matsumoto T, Shinohara M. Oxygen availability and motor unit activity in humans. Eur J Appl Physiol 1992; 64 : 552 – 556.

Naito H, Powers SK, Demirel HA, Sugiura T, Dodd SL, Aoki J. Heat stress attenuates skeletal muscle atrophy in hindlimb-unweighted rats. J Appl Physiol 2000; 88 : 359 – 363.

Pierce JR, Clark BC, Ploutz-Snyder LL, Kanaley JA. Growth hormone and muscle function responses to skeletal muscle ischemia. J Appl Physiol 2006; 101 : 1588 – 1595.

Reeves GV, Kraemer RR, Hollander DB, Clavier J, Thomas C, Francois M, Castracane VD. Comparison of hormone responses following light resistance exercise with partial vascular occlusion and moderately difficult resistance exercise without occlusion. J Appl Physiol 2006; 101 : 1616 – 1622.

Reid MB. Role of nitric oxide in skeletal muscle: synthesis, distribution and functional importance. Acta Physiol Scand 1998; 162 : 401 – 409.

Schuelke M, Wagner KR, Stolz LE, Hubner C, Riebel T, Komen W, Braun. T, Tobin JF, Lee SJ. Myostatin mutation associated with gross muscle hypertrophy in a child. N Engl J Med 2004; 350 : 2682 – 2688.

Senf SM, Dodd SL, McClung JM, Judge AR. Hsp70 overexpression inhibits NF-kappaB and Foxo3a transcriptional activities and prevents skeletal muscle atrophy. FASEB J 2008; 22 : 3836 – 3845.

Sumide T, Sakuraba K, Sawaki K, Ohmura H, Tamura Y. Effect of resistance exercise training combined with relatively low vascular occlusion. J Sci Med Sport 2007.

Takano H, Morita T, Iida H, Asada K, Kato M, Uno K, Hirose K, Matsumoto A , Takenaka K, Hirata Y, Eto F, Nagai R, Sato Y, Nakajima T. Hemodynamic and hormonal responses to a short-term low-intensity resistance exercise with the reduction of muscle blood flow . Eur J Appl Physiol 2005; 95 : 65 – 73.

Takarada Y, Nakamura Y, Aruga S, Onda T, Miyazaki S, Ishii N. Rapid increase in plasma growth hormone after low-intensity resistance exercise with vascular occlusion. J Appl Physiol 2000; 88 : 61 – 65.

References (cont)

Takarada Y, Takazawa H, Sato Y, Takebayashi S, Tanaka Y, Ishii N. Effects of resistance exercise combined with moderate vascular occlusion on muscular function in humans. J Appl Physiol 2000; 88 : 2097 - 2106.

Takarada Y, Takazawa H, Ishii N. Application of vascular occlusion diminish disuse atrophy of knee extensor muscles. Med Sci Sports Exerc 2000; 32 : 2035 - 2039.

Uematsu M, Ohara Y, Navas JP, Nishida K, Murphy TJ, Alexander RW, Nerem RM, Harrison DG. Regulation of endothelial cell nitric oxide synthase mRNA expression by shear stress . Am J Physiol 1995; 269 : C1371 - C1378.

Victor RG, Seals DR. Reflex stimulation of sympathetic outflow during rhythmic exercise in humans. Am J Physiol 1989; 257 : H2017 - H2024.

Wang X, Proud CG. The mTOR pathway in the control of protein synthesis. Physiology (Bethesda) 2006; 21 : 362 - 369.

Yarasheski KE, Campbell JA, Smith K, Rennie MJ, Holloszy JO, Bier DM. Effect of growth hormone and resistance exercise on m muscle growth in young men. Am J Physiol 1992; 262 : E261 - E267.

Z-Health. (n.d.). http://zhealtheducation.com/

www.ingramcontent.com/pod-product-compliance
Lightning Source LLC
Chambersburg PA
CBHW072018280526
45788CB00007B/2601